How to

Overcome

osteoporosis

By

Lucy Becker

TABLE OF CONTENTS

*Those who are susceptible to vitamin K2 deficiency

*How much vitamin K2 should I consume each day

*vitamin D3

*The ideal set of bones are here.

Introduction

Osteoporosis is a medical disorder that causes bones to become less dense, which can make them brittle and more likely to break. The Greek words "osteo" (which means bone) and "poros," which means porous or spongy, are the origin of the word "osteoporosis." Our bodies naturally lose bone density as we age, but in those who have osteoporosis, this loss happens considerably more quickly, leaving them with fragile bones that are more prone to breaking. Both men and women can develop osteoporosis, but women are more likely to do so, particularly after menopause. Additional factors that increase your risk of developing osteoporosis include having the condition in your family, being underweight, leading a sedentary lifestyle, smoking, drinking too much alcohol, and having certain medical problems or taking medications that harm your bones. Because osteoporosis typically goes unnoticed until a bone fractures, it is frequently referred to as a "silent illness." Hip, spine, and wrist fractures are the most frequent types of fractures in patients with osteoporosis. Osteoporosis is treated with drugs that decrease bone loss, increase bone density, and lower the risk of fractures, as well as lifestyle adjustments like weight-bearing exercise and a calcium- and vitamin D-rich diet. Frail, brittle, and weak bones associated with osteoporosis increase the risk of fractures. Osteoporosis is a systemic skeletal disorder characterized by low bone density cell mass, micro-architectural degradation of bone tissue that results in bone fragility, and an increased risk of fractures. In senior persons, it is the most common cause of a broken bone. Among the bones that are prone to breaking include the forearm bones, the hip, and the vertebrae in the spine. Typically, a broken bone doesn't show any symptoms until it actually happens. Bones can weaken to the point where they can break on their own or with minimal exertion. As the broken bone heals, the patient could continue to experience pain and lose some of their ability to carry out regular chores. Several conditions or treatments, including alcoholism, anorexia, and hyperthyroidism, have the potential to result in osteoporosis. Many medicines speed up the rate of bone loss. Insufficient exercise and smoking are additional risk factors.

Prevention

What immediately comes to mind when you consider bone health and the best supplements to assist it? Surely calcium and vitamin D? But what if I told you that vitamin K2 and calcium might be a good combination? Without a doubt, calcium is necessary, but there is a negative aspect to it that most people are unaware of. We must direct calcium toward the bones;

simply taking calcium is insufficient. Our soft tissues, such as arteries and joints, are the last places we want calcium because it can increase the risk of heart attacks, strokes, and discomfort. If we take calcium carelessly and don't pay attention to where it travels, it will end up there. Another well-known mineral that is well-known in the research community is vitamin D, which is now even being given for hospitalized patients. Fall prevention strategies might also include vitamin D. The doses may range from 1,000 IUs per day to 50,000 IUs per week. The absorption of calcium is enhanced by vitamin D. More calcium will be absorbed if you take it alongside vitamin D. That might sound nice, but if you don't have enough vitamin K2 available, the calcium will wind up in the wrong places. Vitamin K2 stimulates osteocalcin, a protein that binds calcium to bone, as well as matrix

GLA, a protein that removes calcium from soft tissues. In order to direct your calcium if you have a lot of it, you need vitamin K2. Consider parking attendants at big events; they direct you where to park your vehicle. Where to put calcium is indicated by K2. It doesn't matter how much calcium you have; what matters is where it ends up. Here are some suggestions for maintaining strong bones without increasing your risk of heart attack.

Calcium should be given first priority in this case so that K2 and D3 can function properly.

 Salmon with soft bones, broccoli, dried beans and peas, sesame seeds, green leafy vegetables, and dairy for those who can tolerate it are all good sources of omega-3 fatty acids. A comprehensive list of calcium-rich foods is also included in the Dietary Guidelines, Only take 500 mg of calcium supplements each day. **MK-7**, a kind of **vitamin K2**, is a daily allowance of up to 300 mcg. *Natto*, a *fermented soy* product, *gouda, edam cheese*, and *butter* from grass-fed cows are food sources of *vitamin K2*. It is okay to take up to *50 mcg of vitamin K2* if you are taking coumadin, but you should always consult with your doctor before taking supplements. Although it is safe to take *1000 IUs of vitamin D* every day and some people require *50,000 IUs per week*, you should first have your levels checked and consult a doctor before taking excessive dosages of the vitamin. Your levels should be examined every year or two, and any vitamin D supplements you take should be in the **D3 (_cholecalciferol_)** form rather than the D2 (ergocalciferol) type. Additionally, magnesium aids in the conversion of vitamin D into its active form. A lack of magnesium exacerbates improper calcification, which results in more calcium entering your soft tissues. **_Vitamin K2_** is the nutrient you want to focus on the most when it comes to bone health. Calcium only serves a useful purpose when it is properly targeted, and **vitamin K2** is the bow that propels **calcium** into the bone. It's very challenging to include all three in a single diet. Therefore, the ideal choices for supplements should include all three components.

Simple strategies for overcoming osteoporosis.

Nutrition: Both vitamins are fat-soluble and work together to assist your body break down calcium by turning on beneficial proteins. **While vitamin D3** increases your ability to absorb calcium, **vitamin K2** determines how that calcium will be utilized. The three key components that encourage bone formation are a diet high in calcium, **vitamin K2**, and *vitamin D*. Even though *vitamin D3* has the ability to start a number of critical biological processes, *vitamin K2* is necessary for their completion and manifestation. Regular resistance and weight-bearing workouts can aid in the development and maintenance of strong bones. however without these essential nutrients in your diet, you wouldn't be able to develop bone, especially when a fracture occurred. When you have osteoporosis, when your bones are fragile and look little, *calcium, vitamin K2, and vitamin D3* are the most effective and crucial elements. These three nutrients support the maintenance of strong bones, teeth, and muscles. It promotes heart health and increases bone mass in cases of postmenopausal osteoporosis. The risk of cardiovascular harm is decreased by *vitamin K2. Vitamin K2* helps the bone collect calcium from blood arteries and transform it into bone tissues by activating the bone-forming protein osteocalcin in the bone. The body can absorb calcium with the aid of *vitamin D3*. It both addresses and averts bone disorders.It is difficult to find diets that have these three in single portions, which is why taking a supplement that contains these three elements is the best way to incorporate them into your diets. *Calcium*, *vitamin K2*, *and vitamin D3* are the best and key components if you want to eliminate osteoporosis, and you must take it in a single pill.

Bone health

The bone matrix contains cells called osteoblasts and osteoclasts that are responsible for breaking down and building up bone in an ongoing remodeling process. Osteoblasts secrete a protein called osteocalcin into the blood which, when activated by *vitamin K2*, binds to *calcium* and transports it from the blood and into the bones. **_Osteoblast_** then integrated this **_calcium_** into the **_bone matrix_**, increasing the bone's mineral density and strength. As part of the remodeling cycle, osteoclasts remove old or damaged bone so that it can be replaced with new cells. As we age, this process of regeneration naturally slows, making bones lighter, more porous and therefore more susceptible to fractures. High levels of uncarboxylated osteocalcin as a result of inadequate *vitamin K2 and D3* intake at any stage of life produce similar effects to the natural aging process.

The researchers concluded that the combination of *vitamins D3 and K2* can significantly increase total BMD and decrease undercarboxylated osteocalcin, and that the effects are more favorable when the two are used in combination. The conclusions we can draw from this body of evidence are clear. The perfect pair combine to increase bone strength and density, suggesting that supplementation with **vitamins D3 and K2** along with **calcium** could help to reduce the risk of fractures and bone loss in older individuals while also supporting the development of strong bones in children. Bone health refers to the overall condition of the skeletal system, which is made up of bones, cartilage, and other connective tissues. Strong and healthy bones are important for maintaining overall health and preventing various conditions such as osteoporosis, fractures, and bone deformities. There are several factors that can affect bone health, including genetics, nutrition, physical activity, and lifestyle habits such as smoking and alcohol consumption. Adequate intake of calcium, vitamin D, and other important nutrients is essential for maintaining strong bones, while regular exercise, especially lifting & weight-bearing exercises, can help strengthen bones and prevent bone loss. To maintain good bone health, it's also important to avoid smoking, limit alcohol intake, and take steps to prevent falls, which can lead to fractures. Women and older adults are particularly at risk for bone-related conditions, so they should be especially vigilant about maintaining good bone health. Regular check-ups with a healthcare provider can help identify any potential problems early on and allow for prompt treatment.

Calcium

Calcium is a mineral that is necessary for keeping bones strong. Osteoporosis, a condition marked by fragile bones, can be brought on by a diet deficient in calcium. Along with regular exercise, a healthy calcium intake can help prevent osteoporosis and preserve strong bones throughout life. For adults, a daily calcium intake of 1000–1200 mg is advised. Dairy products, leafy greens, and fortified foods like orange juice and tofu are all excellent sources of calcium.

facts on vitamin K2

The preservation of bone health and potential prevention of osteoporosis are both facilitated by vitamin K2, it has been shown. Vitamin K2 is a fat-soluble vitamin that is essential to the body's blood clotting process and aids in the activation of proteins involved in bone formation and maintenance. Vitamin K2 also assists in directing calcium to the bones. Menaquinone (MK), the most prevalent kind of vitamin K2, is a compound that is present in both fermented foods and animal products. The regulation of calcium deposition in bones is another function of vitamin K2, which is crucial for maintaining bone health.

Studies have suggested that vitamin K2 may help prevent arterial calcification and reduce the risk of heart disease.

Some research also suggests that vitamin K2 may have anti-inflammatory properties and could potentially be beneficial in the prevention and treatment of certain types of cancer. Vitamin K2 deficiency is relatively rare but may occur in people with malabsorption disorders or those who are taking certain medications that interfere with vitamin K absorption.

Although the optimal daily dose of vitamin K2 for adults has not yet been determined, several sources propose a range of 45–185 mcg per day for adults. Natto, cheese, and sauerkraut are examples of foods high in vitamin K2, as are animal products like liver, egg yolks, and butter from grass-fed cows. When taken in the authorized dosages, vitamin K2 is usually regarded as being safe, although large doses may have undesirable side effects including flushing or perspiration.

Large doses of vitamin K2 may interfere with the efficiency of blood-thinning drugs like warfarin, so those who take these should be careful. For healthy bones, it is necessary. Some studies suggest that increasing vitamin K2 intake can improve bone density and reduce fracture risk in individuals with osteoporosis. The K vitamin family is an essential part of the nutritional web needed to maintain healthy biological functions. There are 12 distinct forms of the vitamin K molecule, all of which are categorized as fat-soluble vitamins. In this book, we'll focus on the two forms of vitamin K2 that are most frequently present in human diets, even though each has a slightly different effect on the body.

K2 MK-4

Any supplement should contain some Vitamin K2 MK-4 since this is the form of the vitamin that is most active in the body. The fact that MK-4 K2 has a brief plasma half-life could be one issue, though. In other words, it leaves the blood swiftly after consumption. Does this imply that vitamin K2 MK-4 supplements are less efficient? Due to its speedy uptake by tissues, organs, and the brain, vitamin K2 (MK-4) should be immediately eliminated from the circulation. MK-4 pills are therefore still effective despite having a short plasma half-life. MK-4 is a molecule that is stored in the pancreas, arteries, and even salivary glands. Although ingestion of animal products makes up a reasonably easy way to receive MK-4, it only accounts for a small fraction of the total vitamin K2 intake. Supporting heart and bone health is the principal application of MK-4.

K2 MK-7

is the least naturally available and most bioactive member of the vitamin K family. Specifically identified fermented foods, like natto cheese, contain K2 MK-7. This nutrient is therefore severely lacking in the diets of the majority of Western consumers. This raises serious concerns because the molecule is crucial for controlling calcium metabolism. Both consumer brands and manufacturers of dietary supplements are learning more about the uses and significance of vitamin K. But most people are still unaware of the advantages vitamin K2 MK-7 can provide, both on its own and in combination with vitamin D3, a molecule already well-known for its health-supporting qualities.

I constantly suggest obtaining Vitamin K2 from food sources as a long-term strategy. However, you might need to take Vitamin K2 supplements if you can't eat enough K2 rich foods or if you have a specific medical condition. Before selecting a vitamin K2 supplement, you should be aware that they vary.

Those who are susceptible to vitamin K2 deficiency

K-vitamin status in children is associated with the development of robust and healthy bones, according to population-based studies and clinical trials. According to a 2008 study, stronger and denser bones were produced in children whose vitamin-K level was improved over a two-year period.

The same group of researchers demonstrated a year later that a small dose of **_vitamin K2 MK-7_** supplementation had enhanced activated osteocalcin, which is a protein that helps create bone, in prepubertal children who were in good health. blood samples from 110 healthy volunteers, including several children and adults, were analyzed in a study that was published in 2012 and involved the participants. By evaluating the levels of circulating inactive MGP and inactive osteocalcin, two proteins related to heart and bone health, respectively, the researchers determined the biomarkers that represented the participants' Vitamin K2 status. According to the study's findings,

MK-7 supplementation had the greatest effects on kids and adults who had the most severe Vitamin K2 deficiencies. The greatest vitamin K2 deficiency was seen in children (and adults over 40, who may benefit from MK-7 supplementation to increase their vitamin k2 status.

How much vitamin K2 should I consume each day

Adult vitamin K2 dosage:

A typical dose is between 100 and 300 mcg per day. For some situations, daily doses of up to 600 mcg may be required.

Children should have 45 mcg of vitamin K2 daily if they are under the age of 12.

Vitamin K2 dosage for osteoporosis: If you have osteoarthritis, your daily requirement may range from 200 mcg to 600 mcg.

K2 manufactured in Norway, America, or Japan is preferred due to its better quality requirements.

vitamin D3

Cholecalciferol, often known as vitamin D3, is a fat-soluble vitamin that is essential for immune system and overall health as well as bone health. The body must be able to absorb calcium and phosphorus in order for them to build strong bones. Fatty fish, egg yolks, and fortified foods like milk are all good food sources of vitamin D3, which the body can also make when exposed to sunlight. A lack of vitamin D3 can cause rickets, osteoporosis, and other health issues. Numerous advantages of vitamin D3 have been demonstrated, including the promotion of bone health, support of a healthy inflammatory response, immune system support, and maintenance of already-normal blood pressure levels. Because of this, some people believe that the "sunshine vitamin" is the most significant vitamin in the body. You might not be aware that this nutrient is also regarded as a hormone. This is due to the fact that **vitamin D3** has receptors in almost all of our body's cells, can be produced by our bodies spontaneously in reaction to sunlight, and can function as a signaling molecule. Most significantly, it improves calcium delivery by enhancing calcium absorption through intestinal walls. In fact, when vitamin D3 is present, calcium absorption increases to 40–50% from the food we eat, compared to only 10-15% when vitamin D3 is absent.

What are some excellent vitamin D3 sources?

Although sunlight is healthy for us, we must take care not to get too much of it. Because of this, daily supplementation with vitamin D3 is the most effective strategy to maintain healthy levels. The largest concentrations of *vitamin D3* can also be found in *animal products; lean seafood options include salmon, swordfish, white fish, and tuna. White meats and hard boiled eggs* are additional vitamin *D3-rich foods.* The highest vitamin D-containing foods for vegans are mushrooms, especially portobello mushrooms.

The ideal set of bones are here.

So how can vitamin D3 and vitamin K2 complement one another? Calcium from your intestines is transported into the blood by **vitamin D3**. The next step is handled by **vitamin K2**, which then directs the calcium to your bones. Consider calcium as a baton, and vitamins D3 and K2 as runners in a relay game of the same name. Both vitamins have many advantages when taken separately, but you need also take ***vitamin D3*** and ***vitamin K2*** supplements to get the most ***calcium***. A little molecule called ***vitamin D*** is able to enter and go to the nucleus of any cell (where vital genetic information is stored). It engages with the promoter regions of human cells, which "decide" whether a gene should be turned on or off. As a result, there is an increase in the creation of the particular protein that the gene is in charge of encoding. Control areas in a variety of cell types interact with **vitamin D3**, as well as **vitamin K2**. Osteocalcin (OC) and matrix Gla protein are two of the most well-known examples of these vitamin K-dependent proteins (**VKDPs**) (**MGP**). However, alone, **vitamin D3** can only express these calcium-binding proteins in their inactive or uncarboxylated state.

Vitamin D3 molecules can promote the expression of these calcium-binding proteins. This makes it difficult for the body to control how calcium from the intestines is incorporated, which could result in decreased bone mass, an increased risk of fracture, and the calcification of arteries and other soft tissues. A sufficient intake of vitamin K2 supports the efficient carboxylation *of OC and MGP* proteins, which in turn aids in the body's ability to bind calcium to bones while maintaining blood levels at the proper levels to prevent vascular calcification. Scientists now refer to the interaction between **vitamins K2 and D3** as a true "synergy" because it may have so many positive effects. When the two molecules work together, they can accomplish more beneficial things than they could do separately. With that in mind, let's examine the particular health areas where this ideal duo provides the most notable advantages for enhanced health and wellbeing.

Can you take vitamin D3 without K2?

It won't hurt to take these two supplements separately, but it will save you time to take them together. The only real consideration to keep in mind is taking vitamin D3 without taking any vitamin K, because if you have a high level of vitamin D3 without enough vitamin K, the calcium might not transfer to the bones properly and instead end up in the vascular tissue. This is because vitamin K is required to activate proteins that concentrate calcium to bones, such as matrix GLA and osteocalcin to the Bone where it's needed most and not to the arteries but before you take this two key supplement make you you are consuming diets rich in calcium and because there is no reason taking the two supplement without calcium, it's would be a good idea if you can take supplement that have all this three element for best possible results on your bone.

How much K2 should I take with D3?

Because vitamin D makes vitamin K2 necessary in the body, taking a vitamin D3 pill without it can have severe consequences.

In terms of collaboration, vitamin K2 is the natural partner of vitamin D3. Respecting D3's ability to significantly improve calcium absorption is the first step in understanding the genius of this combination. Recent studies have revealed that consuming too much calcium by itself might be hazardous to the body. The extra calcium needs to be used properly or it could end up in the wrong locations and lead to illness. Another regulating function of vitamin K that keeps bones appropriately mineralized with a strong protein matrix is the carboxylation of osteocalcin.

Moreover, activated osteocalcin activates adiponectin, a powerful activator of fat metabolism that aids in maintaining a healthy weight. It is thought that the majority of antibiotics used in animal feedlots today are making their way into consumers' stomachs, severely disrupting the good bacteria that convert vitamin K into its active form. (Thus, a deficiency in vitamin K may be a factor in the current obesity epidemic!) Coronary and carotid artery calcification can be avoided by activating the vascular GMP protein. This explains why frequent vitamin K users see a heart disease reduction of more than 50%. Bone spurs may not form if the same protein is consumed. Hence, rather than the other way around, vitamin K promotes "strong bones and soft arteries," which help us age better. Strong evidence supports vitamin K's extraordinary capacity to lower cancer risk, just like vitamin

D3 does. *Men can statistically cut their risk of prostate cancer by 60% by taking vitamin K2 mk7 (a naturally occurring long-acting version of K2) at a dose of 45 mcg per day, for instance.* It is just one of the many cancer risks that are highly considerably decreased by consistent K2 consumption. We have determined that it is reasonable to combine the safety and efficacy of this potent pair as we investigate the therapeutic potential of greater dosages of vitamin D3 at the **_Reagan Health center_**. We advise 100 mcg of K2 mk7 for every 2,500–5,000 units of D3 that are suggested and tested for in order to be safe and avoid the unwarranted calcification that higher doses of D3 alone might result in.

SUMMARY

Studies indicate that having these three elements in one pill with a large meal or source of fat can significantly increase absorption of calcium to the Bone.

Many people prefer to take supplements rather than diets that have all these three elements first thing in the morning. Not only is it often more convenient, but it's also easier to remember your vitamins in the morning than later in the day.

This is especially true if you're taking multiple supplements, as it can be challenging to stagger supplements or medications throughout the day. For this reason, it may be best to get in the habit of taking these supplements that have **calcium**, **vitamin k2 and D3** with a nutritious breakfast. However, there's limited research on whether taking it at night or in the morning may be more effective. The most important steps are to fit all these three elements into your routine and take it consistently to ensure maximum effectiveness. Try taking it alongside breakfast or with a bedtime food as long as it doesn't interfere with your sleep. The key is to find what works for you and stick with it to ensure you're meeting your need for these three elements. It's crucial to consult your doctor to create a customized plan to treat and prevent osteoporosis based on your unique requirements and current health state.